MW01118717

FOR THE MOMENT-ALZHEIMER'S DISEASE

Janet B. Gundlach

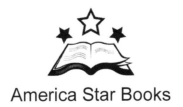

America Star Books

© 2014 by Janet B. Gundlach.
All rights reserved. No part of this book may be reproduced, stored in a retrieval system or transmitted in any form or by any means without the prior written permission of the publishers, except by a reviewer who may quote brief passages in a review to be printed in a newspaper, magazine or journal.

First printing

America Star Books has allowed this work to remain exactly as the author intended, verbatim, without editorial input.

Softcover 9781632492937
PUBLISHED BY AMERICA STAR BOOKS, LLLP
www.americastarbooks.com

Dedicated to my wonderful Husband, Chuck
who was the best Son to his Mother and to
our children and grandchildren who loved
their Grandmother and Great-Grandmother
with their whole hearts.

TABLE OF CONTENTS

PREFACE

Alzheimer's is a "progressive, degenerative brain disease with gradual onset". It is the death of nerve cells in the brain. When enough of those cells die, symptoms of the disease appear. Alzheimer's disease is a type of dementia that causes a steady decline in memory, thinking and behavior. The disease progresses over 2-20 years and varies considerable from person to person. After age 5, the likelihood of developing the disease doubles every 5 years. After age 85 progression is most rapid.

It is the second most feared disease after cancer. An estimated 5.4 million Americans are living with it, and there's no cure!

U.S. health authorities are recommending that doctors diagnose the risk of developing Alzheimer's disease before people develop full-blown dementia.

The recommendations are aimed at helping patients and their families prepare financially, logistically and emotionally for the disease, which can require years of intensive, expensive care.

As we age we seem to forget from time to time. When my husband's Mom started to forget, we just thought she was going through the aging process. At age 82, Mom was forgetting all the important things to live a normal life.

This book is meant to help "CAREGIVERS" figure out what is happening to their parents or loved one as they start out with Alzheimer's disease and progress through it. In the eight years that "Mom" had been going through the disease we have learned a lot on our own and with the help of many other people.

I hope this book will give you the knowledge and help you need to guide you in the right, safe direction of your family member.

IN THE BEGINNING

Everything can seem just fine in your life until one day your loved one starts to forget. I don't mean just forget "FOR THE MOMENT", but starting to forget all the important things. My husband, Chuck's "Mom" lived in her own home for 57 years and for the last seventeen of those years without his "DAD", who died of lung cancer. She never wanted to bother us unless she needed our advice or when something needed to be fixed in her home or her car needed to be looked at, as we worked and were raising four children. She tried to do things on her own. She was independent and drove until she was 85 years old. The signs of Alzheimer's started when she was 82 years of age, but we had no idea what was happening to her.

When Mom was 82, her tax accountant said he was retiring and he could not do her taxes anymore. Mom told Chuck, so he decided he could just go over the last year's tax forms and do it himself. We never asked Mom what monies she had and she never discussed it with us. We always thought she had enough money to pay her bills and then some. She had no mortgage or car payment. As family members age, there should be conversation about what they want to do, where they want to live and how much they have to live on for the rest of their lives. We should realize that anything can happen to us and we should be prepared.

Mom started selling her life insurance policies and we did not know why. When Chuck started doing her taxes that next year, he started to ask her questions about why she cashed in her life insurance policy. She was using the money from her insurance policies to pay for property taxes. The property taxes started to go up high, but she did not realize she could get a Senior Tax Freeze on them. Chuck was able to get her property taxes reduced.

She has needed a new car for many years, but we thought she just did not want to give up the car because Dad bought it and they rode together in it. It was really because she knew she did not have the money and didn't want to tell us.

As time went by, Mom would leave her bills on the kitchen table because she could not remember how to pay them anymore. Chuck took charge of paying her bills.

When Chuck retired he was able to take his Mom to the hair dresser in town every Saturday. We lived one hour away from her. Mom always had her very thick, beautiful hair done every week.

Since Mom lived in her own home, she used to be physically able to keep it up, but now she did not remember to do it. She always kept a clean, spotless home. She would always have everything put away except the bills on the table in the kitchen. Her dishes were always washed after she ate, but she started to forget that she did them.

She would walk down 4 stairs to the landing in her home and then 7 stairs to the basement to do her laundry, but would always forget that she put the clothes in the washer or didn't dry the clothes. When we came on our visits, I would check the washing machine and dryer to make sure she got the laundry. She stopped washing her sheets and towels, too. It was hard for her not to be able to do what she once did especially when she took pride in herself for being self-sufficient.

We would shop for her meals now. First we tried frozen prepared foods, but she never liked frozen foods. She always loved broccoli, brussels sprouts, fresh bread, lamb chops and pork tenderloin. She would bake the lamb chops and pork tenderloin in the oven. All that stopped as she could not remember any more.

I spoke with our neighbor one day about our Mom and she said she buys already prepared fresh food from a local grocery store, Cuputos, and brings them to her college children. Mom had a wonderful store that she use to shop in called Happy Foods and they had prepared food. Mom was good about heating up her food in the microwave.

She always had cereal for breakfast so Chuck made sure she had a few boxes on hand and fresh milk with a good date on it. She had bananas on her cereal so we would bring her bananas twice a week when we would bring the meals. Lunch could be a toasted muffin with ham and cheese on it. She loved her tea so she would heat her water in a very loud whistling tea kettle. One day, however, Chuck's sister called him and said: "Mom told me she burnt the tea kettle".

When the cold weather came, Mom would always turn on the gas stove burner and "warm her hands" and keep it on until the kitchen got warmer. It was a "habit" she did all he life! We knew she did it and we kept telling her not to do it!

Her pantry had to be cleaned out now as she had old soup, flour, sugar and spices that hadn't been used for quite a while.

Now we were cleaning her home, doing her bills and banking. Chuck went to the bank with Mom and had them add his name to her accounts. We would do her laundry, grocery shopping and ordering her pills, sorting her pills and calling her at least two to three times a day to make sure she had eaten and taken her pills. I kept a list of all of Mom's medication and all her surgeries and shots, in my wallet in case we had to take her to the hospital for an emergency. We took her blood pressure every week.

We had a calendar for all her Doctor Appointments, hair appointments including hair cuts and permanents so we could keep scheduling them when needed. We became her "social secretary" as her friends from "High School" would make a date once a month to take her to lunch with them. Mom's dear friend would pick her up and bring her to Bible Study at her church each week. She even had Dad's friends from Lions Club pick her up and take her to lunch, too. We had to make sure we called her to tell her to get dressed and be ready by the time they told her. We were thankful she still was able to write the times down, but needed us to remind her.

In the summer time Mom loved to have beautiful geraniums in the window boxes on the outside of the garage. Mom now forgot to water them. The following year we put in "FAKE" flowers so we did not have to worry about them dying and to make her home looked lived in!! The landscaper had been coming every week in the summer ever since Dad died to cut and trim her lawn.

Mom had a wonderful neighbor across the street who would always check in on her. Mom would call her a lot whenever she had a problem. WE WERE VERY THANKFUL FOR HER. If she could help her that was great, otherwise Mom would call us. One day her neighbor saw us and said: "Your Mom is really forgetting!" Some of our good friends told us they helped their neighbors who were in their 90's and would check on them and shop for them daily if they needed anything. These people were still able to take care of themselves, but had a hard time getting out because they did not drive anymore or were handicapped. When Dad was alive, Mom did this for her 93 year old Aunt who lived a few miles from her.

By now the decisions were becoming very hard for us to make for all of Mom's needs.

CAREGIVERS

WE REALIZED WHEN MOM WAS FORGETTING A LOT IN HER HOME THAT WE WERE HER CAREGIVERS!

Your parents brought you up. Now it's your turn to care of them—which will bring unique challenges, and very possibly some surprises.

It has become time to parent the parent. We are the sandwich generation. Caregivers report having to give up exercise, vacations, and social activities with no free weekends. At the same time though, many women say that it's a life-enriching responsibility and that there are lots of ways for you to meet your parents' needs and your own.

According to the Pew Research Center, one out of every eight Americans ages 40-60 is raising a child as well as caring for a parent at home. Seven million to ten million adults are caring for their aging parents from long distance. One Third of those caregivers are men. While I have 6 sisters and 2 brothers, we were all able to have our Mother live with us for a certain period of time after we sold her home in Florida. When she got very weak, our sister, the nurse, was able to have my Mom live with her until she died.

Chuck's two sisters lived farther away and would come a few times a year to see Mom. We were very fortunate to have our children and my sister help us out with Chuck's Mom when she lived in her home and then at the Retirement Center because it became necessary to watch over her every day.

If siblings live close by they can take turns taking their loved ones to Doctors appointments and food shopping, etc. It helps to designate different jobs so they get used to it on a regular basis.

In April of 2003, Mom had a stress test and had blockage in her left leg. She had several tests for her clogged arteries.

January, 2007, Mom called her neighbor next door because she was very anxious, shaky and nervous. Chuck and I went to pick her up and take her home after calling the Doctor. Mom wanted us to take her to see her Doctor. We took her to the Doctor and he wanted us to take her to our house for observation. Mom was starting to forget taking her medication. Her blood pressure was very high. After we got to our home, Mom was very upset and paced the floor. She said: "I Want To Go Home!" We gave her Xanax medication to calm her down. "For The Moment" this was the first time ever that Mom got very angry so it was sad to see this happening to her. We did take her home. We also knew she couldn't live alone any more. Chuck's sisters said that Mom had gotten angry at them, too, when she went to visit them.

One Sunday in July, 2007, Mom was at her church and got very sweaty, cold and had neck pain. We thought we better take her to the hospital. She had an angiogram and had blockage in her right coronary artery. She was put on new medication, Plavix, a prescription used to treat high blood pressure and angina. With all her heart problems we wondered if that was the start of something happening to her brain cells, too.

We received a brochure in the mail from a Retirement Center. It listed all the things Mom was going through and used the words "ALZHEIMER"S DISEASE". It really helped us focus on the decisions we needed to make for Mom now that she was not capable of doing it herself. I am going to try to guide you into this information so that it might help you better understand what is happening to your loved one and what you can do to help them.

ALZHEIMER"S DISEASE

One of the worst things about Alzheimer's Disease is the way it sneaks up on its victims. By the time the first signs appear, it may be too late for lifestyle therapies like staying mentally and socially active. It effects more than 5 million Americans and a number that will grow to 13.4 million by 2050. There is no cure as of this date.

Alzheimer's is driven by genes. The disease is thought to be caused by a buildup of protein-based plaques in the brain. Early-Stage Alzheimer's can start in your late 50's and progress in the years ahead. Mom's Alzheimer's started in her early 80's. Early onset numbers are rising.

SIGNS OF ALZHEIMER'S DISEASE
Increased confusion, disorientation or inability to concentrate.
Deteriorating hygiene or pride in appearance.
Erratic or inappropriate behavior changes.
Emotional problems, depression or stress that linger and persist.
Signs of insufficient nutrition, dehydration, weight loss or bad diet (like a poorly stocked pantry, expired items in the refrigerator or signs of not cooking/eating healthy).
Inability to manage money, bills not getting paid or mail piling up.
Inability to manage medications.

Unclean or unsafe living environment including slippery sidewalks, dirty dishes in the sink or stress over the burden of household chores.

Loneliness or house-bound "cabin fever" especially in winter.

Millions of people suffer from Alzheimer's disease and treatment options are "limited".

Existing drugs may mask symptoms for a time but do nothing to stop the relentless downward progression of Alzheimer's.

Mom's primary Doctor was her Heart Doctor. She would have a check-up every year and was on medicine for her heart and cholesterol medicine. She did have a mild heart attack in 1991. We asked Mom's doctor if ARICEPT medication, used to treat mild, moderate and severe Alzheimer's patients would help her and he said it was worth trying. We don't think at her age of 86 it helped her that much. We asked him what else we could do and he said :"LET HER LIVE HER LIFE"! AND WE DID JUST THAT TO THE BEST OF OUR ABILITY!

We really, really tried hard to let Mom keep her independence. We told the doctor, Mom really slept very well and he said: "GOD'S BLESSING TO SLEEP MORE!" You will eventually need 24-hour-a-day care, but we don't have enough caretakers and facilities.

As of this date Hospitals and Senior Centers and the Private Sectors are starting to build many "MEMORY CARE" facilities.

FEAR

In the middle of the night at 2:30 a.m., we got a call from Mom. She said: "I locked myself in my bedroom. I am frightened". We did not know if she had heard someone or something to be frightened or just frightened. This was the first time we had this call so we got in the car and drove the hour to her home. We kept in communication with her with our cell phone to make sure she did not hear any noises in case someone might be in the home. We were almost positive that she was just frightened. When we got there, we forgot that Mom had a bolted lock on the inside of the door that had no key. WE had to tell her to come unlock the door. She at first, did not want to do that. After coaxing her, she finally came out of her room and unlocked the door.

FEAR is a part of Alzheimer's. My friend's Dad had Dementia and he wold get very angry because he was forgetting. They finally had to put him in a full care facility.

We were afraid to leave Mom alone now, but one of our friends told us about "LIFE ALERT". The company comes to your home and hooks up a device that is connected to the telephone. Mom would wear a pendant around her neck or on her wrist. If she fell or was frightened she would just press the button on the pendant. If she were to hit the button they first would call her to see if she was okay and/or call us. She was pretty secure with this and it gave us a little extra comfort. She had bumped the devise a few times and the service would first call her and ask her if she was okay and she would laugh and say: "Oh Yes, I just bent over and hit it by mistake." There is a monthly fee for this service.

THE BATHROOM

Chuck installed a hand bar in the bath tub area for Mom to hold on to when she got out of the bath tub, but she really didn't like the way it looked! She was still taking a shower at age 84, but not as often. Some caregivers have a special bath tub with a door installed so you can walk into it. There is also a hand-held shower sprayer you can install in the bath tub or shower. A chair can be put in the tub and/or shower also.

Mom would put her feet up to the sink, one at a time, just like her Mom did when she got older, and wash them instead of taking a shower. We told her that was not a safe idea. She would just laugh.

Keeping independent to bathe is very important, but much harder when you do not have a separate shower as it is hard for an older person to lift their legs in and out of the bath tub without falling.

When Mom moved into the retirement home she had a walk-in shower. I would check to see if she used the shower. She was doing this less and less now and we would tell her we weren't leaving until she took a shower. She did not like that but knew we meant well so she did what we said.

We would always check to see if she had toothpaste, a good toothbrush, her eye make-up and face make-up, lotion, hair spray, toilet paper, face soap, scope, etc.

We had made a list of all the brand names Mom used so it was easier for us to replace them. Chuck bought two of each item at a time so we never ran out of them.

THE CAR

At age 85 Mom had passed her driving test, but we really knew she should not drive. How do you tell your parents they can not drive!!! Mom would drive into town a few miles away from where she lived and would attend a Bible Study each week at her church and then would stop for groceries at Happy Foods in town. One day when she got to the church she couldn't remember where she was and our Pastor called us and told us what happened. A friend drove her home and Chuck and I drove to church and got her car. Mom never said a word about the car after that, almost like she knew that was the last time she would drive. A few months later Chuck tried to start the car but the battery was dead. He told his Mom that the car didn't work and he was not getting it fixed. He took the car keys to our home and the car sat in her garage.

MONEY AND THE BILLS

We knew Mom would not be able to stay in her own home, but we did not know when to take action to move her. Some of our friends PANICKED when their parents were going through Alzheimer's. Sometimes things happen so quickly that you only have a few weeks or few days to find a place for your parents.

We had to find all the paper work and then found out everything we needed to know to put Mom's house on the market. Mom did not want to move from her home. We did have her on a waiting list at a Retirement Center called Covenant Village in Northbrook, IL, but nothing was available at the time. This Retirement Center is affiliated with our Church's denomination and we always knew Mom would want to be there as a lot of her friends from her Church lived there.

Chuck and I were driving to Mom's quite often each week now because Mom stopped driving. We still had no idea of any money she had or where she kept all her records. By this time Mom was not able to remember any thing about her paper work or where it was. Chuck and I had to "find" the Wooden Box and File Box with all the paper work in it in her closet. Mom had kept all the checks that had cleared the bank, and statements from way before Dad died 17 1/2 years ago. We started going through everything from Title to the House, the Insurance Policy for the House and anything relating to house expenses. There was her Pension, checking account, insurance for her and the burial information that she had kept from Dad's funeral. We needed to find her records for all her health issues.

We were lucky that Mom was a very neat house keeper. We have heard stories from people who had to clean out their parents homes.

We received a call from the Retirement Home and they said they wanted us to come and visit a studio apartment they had available for Mom. We went the next week and realized we needed to get Mom moved in as soon as possible, talked with Chuck's sisters and we agreed to take it. They said it would take around three months to sell her home and move her into the new home. We were very relieved that we would now get her out of her house.

SELLING THE HOUSE

Another thing for a caregiver to do is to TELL YOUR PARENT THEY HAVE TO SELL THEIR HOME. It had become too dangerous for Mom to live in her home without anyone living with her. Some caregivers have a "live-in" for their parents. We know of people who took out extended health care insurance and it actually does work. We wanted Mom to still be able to be as active as she could at Covenant Village surrounded by a lot of her friends.

At age 85, Mom was still capable of signing documents. Chuck took her to the lawyer and had a POWER OF ATTORNEY document drawn up. This Power of Attorney authorized Chuck to sign any document regarding Mom in case she could not do this. WE WERE ESPECIALLY THANKFUL THAT CHUCK HAD THE POWER OF ATTORNEY WHEN MOM HAD HER STROKE IN 2009. EVERYTHING FELL INTO PLACE WHENEVER CHUCK HAD TO SIGN ANYTHING FOR MOM. HER WILL ALSO NEEDED TO BE REDONE. WE HAD THE ATTORNEY PUT HER WILL INTO A TRUST.

We called our neighbor who is a Realtor and had her find a Realtor in Mom's neighborhood and put Mom's house on the market. The Realtor was very nice and understood Mom's needs. We agreed on a price and

Mom signed the papers, which she did not want to do, but said: "I know I have to do this" with us there. We felt confident that the Realtor could show the house even if Mom was home. She knew Mom had a hard time remembering. The Realtor would always call us before showing the house. The Realtor said she would always be there with the other Realtor so Mom would be comfortable if anyone came into her home. When the Realtor called us to show the house, we would decide if we needed to go and tidy up the house.

A wonderful couple love the house and put a bid on it. This was in June, 2007 The day before we closed the Realtor said that she could not close on a house the day before because something was happening to mortgages. We were thankful the house closed because that weekend the housing market stopped!!! We needed the money from Mom's house to get her into the Retirement Home.

At this writing because of the economy, it is still very difficult for older people to sell their home so they can go into a Retirement Home.

TRAVELING

Because Chuck's sisters lived in North Carolina and Ohio they were not able to help us very much. Ever since Dad died they called Mom every night to make sure she was okay. Once or twice a year Mom was able to still travel via airplane to their homes for a week. His sisters made the arrangements for the flights as Mom was not capable of doing that anymore. We would take her to the airport and had prearranged for a wheelchair for Mom as she had arthritis in her one knee and could not walk long distances. We would make sure Mom got taken care of to her gate.

When Mom was 88, she traveled to Chuck's sisters home and Mom had an "accident" in their home and his sisters decided Mom ha to wear depends. Mom was in a "different environment" and eating "different" kinds of foods so perhaps she couldn't get to the bathroom fast enough. From then on Mom has worn depends, but did not have a lot of accidents and at age 91 she was able to tell us she had to go to the bathroom a lot of the time.

That was also the last time Mom flew in a plane.

THE MOVE FROM THE HOUSE TO THE RETIREMENT HOME

Mom was not capable of making decision about all the things in her home of 57 years. This was one of the hardest things we had to do to move her into the Retirement Home. The 60 days before we moved Mom into her apartment, Chuck and I would spend sleepless nights worrying about the sale of the house, moving, and Mom's health.

Every day we would drive to her house with boxes and start packing up her things. She was moving into a studio apartment so we could not take a lot of furniture. We visualized how she would like her apartment. We took her credenza that was Dad's, and matching night stand with a lamp, her TV cabinet and TV with the REMOTE that she was familiar with, her recliner, two chairs, table lamp, love seat and her beautiful breakfront with all her beautiful collections of Lladros and special gifts from friends and relatives and her Aunt's treasured pieces inside it. Her Dad's very special chair had a place next to her bed. We were able to take a few big pictures and a small glass table that held her special pictures. Her Hope Chest fit at the end of her bed. The only thing that was new was a twin bed that we bought with her to make sure it was comfortable. We helped her pick out drapes and a matching comforter. Her regular, corded phone was by her bed side and her regular cordless phone, which she was very familiar with, was on a lamp table next to her recliner. She could still use the phone to call us if she had to.

TO MAKE MOM FEEL MORE COMFORTABLE, WE NEEDED TO KEEP EVERYTHING IN HER APARTMENT LOOK LIKE HER SURROUNDINGS THAT WERE IN HER HOUSE. THIS WAS VERY IMPORTANT. With her arthritis in her hands, she needed to have the same lamps that she remembered how to turn on. We tried not to change the environment she was use to so she was comfortable and it was less confusing for her. We copied, in large print, the phone numbers of the front desk, Chuck's phone number and his sisters numbers and laminated it and put it by her phone.

We bought a wonderful 24 inch X 36 inch frame and put pictures of Dad and Mom and all of her Children and Grandchildren and Great-Grandchildren and Brother's family and a picture of their house and a few other fun pictures in it. We hung it in her kitchenette area so she would be reminded of all the love that surrounds her. Dad had carved a small bird 20 years ago and glued it on their kitchen wall that had a mural on it. I was able to glue the little bird inside the frame. We hung a small full length mirror next to the night stand so Mom could look into it when she got dressed.

On the final day when she moved into her new apartment we looked around and saw that it looked like her "mini house". We were SO VERY HAPPY! Mom did not have much emotion about it now, but in our hearts we knew she would be safe there. Every time we left Mom she would follow us out her door and ask: "What do I do now?" We said: "Mom, go back inside your room and watch the news" and she did. She still seemed to sleep through the night.

THE CLOTHES

When we were moving Mom from her house to her apartment, we had to decide which clothes to take with. Mom loved her clothes and had a lot of matching outfits, shoes and purses. I even put "week days", Monday, Tuesday, etc. on door signs like the ones children make with their names on them, and put each one on Mom's matching clothes hangers, but she didn't seem to understand how that worked!!

I went through the latest pictures of Mom with our families and saw what clothes she wore and that helped me. We were very thankful Mom cold still dress herself and comb her hair. I matched up her clothes so that helped her. When we moved Mom it was summer time so I had to take the winter clothes and put them in plastic bags for the second closet. I chose her good shoes and boots. Mom only once wore gym shoes and did not like them, but I took them anyway just in case she would need them. Mom always wore high heels all life and we brought a few pairs with, but she never wore them. We chose her dress coat and every day coat and a few sweaters, gloves and scarf. It was hard getting rid of her mink hat as no one wanted it not even the resale shop. We packed up all the extra clothes and gave them to "the Salvation Army" which Mom had been supporting all her life.

Mom had made hats and bought a lot of hats. She looked beautiful in them. We had used some of her hats for tea parties for our grandchildren. On the last day of clearing out her home and piles of things placed on the sidewalk for "Salvation Army" to pick them up, the hat boxes were "calling me" and I couldn't bear to let them take them so they went in our car and we took them to our home. It was a very hard, sad day to see the house empty. Mom was living at Covenant Village now and we felt it best that she did not come to the house as we were finishing emptying it.

MEDICATION

Mom had been on Aricept medication for a few years now. Aricept is used to treat mild, moderate and severe Alzheimer's patients that could possibly slow the progression of Alzheimer's. We really believed Mom was too far along with Alzheimer's to make a difference, but we thought it might help. It is a medication that really should be started with the onset of Alzheimer's.

She was on Plavix, a medication to help prevent a heart attack.

She was also taking Norvasc, a medication to help control her blood pressure.

Her Doctor had us give Xanax on occasion when she started to get very nervous and anxious after we moved her into the retirement center.

Chuck was purchasing all of Mom's medication now and would put them in "daily reminder" pill dispensers. He would call her three times a day to make sure she got up and ate breakfast, took her pills, got dressed and be ready to go down to the dining room for lunch and dinner.

THE HYGIENE

When Mom was in her home, we noticed she was taking less and less showers, but we thought that in her apartment with just a shower to get in and out of and not a bath tub, she would be taking more showers.

We would check to see if the shower stall was being used and we could tell Mom was not bathing. Chuck and I would say: Before we go home Mom, we are going to wait until you take a shower. She would say that she did not want to get into her pajamas yet, so we said: "Okay, you can put your clothes back on after you shower". I would turn on the shower for her. She was still good about doing that and we made sure she showered several days a week.

She always brushed her teeth every time she ate and would rinse her mouth out with scope. NOTE: Mom never, ever had a cold, cough, flu or any viruses. We were very thankful for that. She still dressed very beautifully and put her make-up on.

Mom always put her glasses, that were in her glass case, in her pocket. When she moved into Covenant Village, she was forgetting her glasses in the dining room. we realized a lot of her pants did not have pockets. We took the pants to the dry cleaning shop and they put pockets in all of her pants. That seemed to help a great deal. Whenever Mom could not find her glasses, we would call the dining room, or craft room and they had them. We put her name inside her glass case.

Mom had Macular Degeneration and we always prayed she would not go blind. She had a wonderful eye specialist that took wonderful care of her eyes.

When she went into full care, the caregivers always put her glasses on her. If Mom took them off, and left them somewhere, there was a drawer by the nurses station and we could retrieve them for her.

Mom did not wear a hearing aid so we were thankful for that. She could not hear very well as she got older but denied that she had a hearing problem.

THE TEST

After Mom had been at Covenant Village for a few months, the nurse was a little concerned about Mom. She said she wanted her to take "The Test" from their Doctor. The Doctor came to Mom's apartment one day. We were not there when she took the tests so do not know totally what went on. We did find the tests on Mom's counter. They were called the "Test Your Memory" (TYM) and the Mini-Mental State Examination (MMSE) tests.

Mom was still able to read with her glasses. Some of the questions were:

Orientation
1. "What is the"(year) (season) (date) (day) (month)?
2. "Where are we?" (state)
Language
3. Ask the patient to recall the 3 items repeated "apple", "table", "penny"

There were 11 questions with a total score of 30. Suggested guideline for determining the severity of cognitive impairment:
Mild:>21, Moderate:>10-20, Severe:>9
Expected decline in MMSE scores in untreated mile to moderate Alzheimer's patient is 2 to 4 points per year.

The doctor said Mom had dementia and that she has had it for some time. She had the inability to learn new techniques and to deal with every day life.

Mom's test results must have been in the "Moderate" range as the nurse recommended that we get help through a SERVICE that was available where helpers would come and take Mom down to the dining room and back again for lunch and dinner. There was a fee for this service. At that time Mom was still able to get her breakfast of cereal, milk, banana and take her pills. She was still taking her pills pretty regularly because Chuck would call her three times a day to remind her to take them.

A Super-simple Alzheimer's Test

According to new Columbia University Research, if you can correctly identify 10 key odors (Menthol, lemon, lilac, leather, clove, strawberry, pineapple, smoke, soap and natural gas), you probably don't have the disease. Researchers say this smell test is so accurate it detected Alzheimer's better than brain scans or genetic testing! (Note: This research seems very hard to believe that I would have to know a lot more about it to see how they came up with this conclusion!)

ANGELS

When Mom moved into her apartment at the Retirement Center, she had a wonderful friend who would come and get her and take her to lunch and dinner. She would drive her to her Church each Sunday. They would eat together and go to the activities together. Mom's apartment complex had several meetings in their social room and her neighbor would always come and take her to the meetings.

It was quite a walk to the dining room and Mom was confused on how to get there alone. Sometimes Chuck would call her to reassure her that she could get there when her friend could not walk with her. We eventually had to pay a "service person" to come get her and bring her to the dining room and back again and sometimes to the craft room. There were other residents that had similar issues that had help, also.

A resident in her building would check every morning to see if the residents put out their "I'M UP" sign on their doors. Mom could not remember to do that although she remembered to get her newspaper most of the time because she always had the paper delivered at her home. The nurse called us and asked us to sign a piece of paper stating that we are okay that Mom does not put her sign out.

My Sister would come and help us with Mom when we would travel to our children and grandchildren's homes or go on vacation.

We realized we were on borrowed time with Mom in her own apartment, but we knew if we had to move her to assisted living we were ready.

After Mom's stroke and her move to full care, many friends came to visit her. Her Church friends, neighbors and family would write notes to her. Even though she could not read them anymore, when Chuck and I came we would read them to her and show her the cards and pictures everyone would send her.

Mom's Pastor and his wife would come regularly to visit with Mom.

We have several friends who are in full care as of this writing. Their children are our children's ages and are working or have their own children to raise. One friend shared with us that her dear friends take a day each week and go visit her Mom and bring cookies and read to her. She says that really helps her out a lot.

"FOR THE MOMENT'" these cards and visits are VERY IMPORTANT!

We are very thankful for all the "ANGELS" that helped us when we needed it the most.

FEAR

Some residents where Mom lived were afraid she would walk out the door and get lost. They felt she was not capable of living alone and needed help. The nurse called and told Chuck that if Mom were to stay there we would have to sign papers stating we take full responsibility if Mom were to leave the building and get lost. He also filled out a policed report from the village that had Mom's name on it and a picture of her. We knew Mom pretty well to realize that she only wanted fresh air and would just put her head out the door on occasion. We would never put Mom in jeopardy of getting hurt. For the 2 1/2 years she lived in her apartment, she never wandered.

After the Doctor gave Mom the Memory Test and evaluated her, the nurse from Covenant Village recommended that we turn off the electric stove in Mom's apartment. Mom was not doing any cooking on her own now so we did unplug the stove.

It was now recommended that we think about moving Mom into assisted living in another building. Chuck and I were now going to her apartment several times a week, bringing her cereal, fresh milk and bananas, doing her laundry, cleaning her apartment, and eating with her in the dining room on occasion. Chuck would still call Mom three times a day for her to take her medicine.

After two and a half years we knew we had to make a new move for her. We did everything in our hearts to help her be independent.

Mom was not getting out of bed in the morning anymore as she did not know what to do. She would leave the drapes closed because she was afraid. She was forgetting a lot more. Chuck would call her and tell her to get up out of bed, get dressed and eat.

Maria Shriver's Dad died in 2011 of Alzheimer's. She said she could not have predicted the profound journey she and her family would make as they tried to understand and cope with the devastating disease. She said she is afraid of getting Alzheimer's—BIG TIME!!

THE STROKE

On December 29th, Chuck called his Mom like he always did early in the morning and there was no answer. He called back every few minutes and no answer. He told me he thinks he should go to see if his Mom was okay. We were thankful that she only lived 20 minutes away. When he opened the door he found his Mom on the floor. He called the nurse and she came and called the Paramedics.

Mom was taken to the hospital and had a lot of tests done. She was paralyzed on the right side. The Doctors said she had a stroke and needed to learn how to eat again with her right hand and try to start walking again. She was not able to communicate. On the third day, she started to walk around the halls of the hospital with a walker. Mom never had a walker until this day. On the fourth day she was released to Brandel Care Center, the rehabilitation center for the residents at Covenant Village.

It was very comforting to know she had a place to go for rehabilitation This is a part of Covenant Villages continuing care. So many of our friends whose parents lived in different Retirement Communities couldn't get their parents into a rehabilitation center when they needed to as they were full and it was frustrating for them.

After three months, we realized Mom could not go back to her apartment. She was not capable of taking care of herself any more. She was in the rehabilitation area due to her stroke and Alzheimer's disease. Chuck and I packed up all of her belongings from her apartment. We had to get rid of all of her furniture except her recliner, bed pillow and comforter. She will share a room with another resident. I had to separate her clothes and take her summer clothes to our house because it was winter and she only had a small wardrobe cabinet, a small dresser that only held a few clothes at a time. There was a TV on the small dresser but Mom did not even watch it. It was another sad day in our lives to move Mom.

Mom would get "bored" just sitting around and would want to go out and sit in the "receptionist area". Note that this rehab center had "lock down" doors where you had to use the "key pad" to get out. Mom could not get dressed by herself anymore or bathe herself. The therapist would come each day to walk Mom down the hall to a therapy center. She would have her meals in a dining room.

Finally, another decision had to be made to put Mom into a "TOTAL LOCK DOWN" facility with 24 hour care. Mom did not get better in rehab and she could not speak very well. "Orchard Court" is a wonderful facility with full care where they had activities all day long. Many of the residents have been there for several years. After we "moved" Mom into this new area we just took one day at at time!!!

Mom was now taken care of by nurses and certified nurses aides (cna's). The facility is right next to the Retirement Center. We moved Mom's pictures of all her family into her room so the nurses and cna's would know what she used to look like and who her family members were when they came to visit. Her Great-Grandchildren would draw pictures and we would put them on her wall.

The nurses and cna's made sure she was dressed with make-up on and her hair combed every day.

Mom always had her hair done once a week by a beautician most of her life so we felt this expense was necessary. A lot of the residents would have their hair just washed and combed after their shower. She would get bathed twice a week. The nurse gave her the medicine she needed. A doctor would come on occasion and check up on her. We did take her to her eye doctor to make sure her vision was as good as it could be so she would not go blind as as she had macular degeneration. We took her back to her favorite Heart Doctor once more for her to see him and to ask him about her medication.

She was on depends and the cna's had a schedule when to take her to the bathroom, but she could sometimes tell the cna's that she had to go to the bathroom when she needed to go. After they dressed her in the morning, the cna's would walk her down to the "dining room/activity room for the whole day. All the residents in Orchard Court would be together all day long unless they were tired and wanted to go to their room.

We could go and sit with Mom when she had her meals or we could reserve a room and bring in our own food and have other family members come, too. We could do crafts with her and sing with her and just sit with her. For one and one-half years Mom lived in Orchard Court so we got to know the residents, their families, the nurses and cna's very well. Mom was 91 years old.

The facility Mom was in was filled with wonderful workers who have a passion to help the Alzheimer's patients, care for them and love them. One resident's wife would come in the morning and stayed with her husband all day long. Another resident's husband would come and hand feed his wife at meal times.

Mom couldn't remember where she was and sometimes asked us abut her house and we said she lives her and she cried. Sometimes she asked what happened to Dad and we told her he died and she cried. She had a hard time speaking. We asked her who we were and she took a while to answer but she usually said our names. A lot of Alzheimer's patients totally forget who their loved ones are and this is very hard for the family!

When we were ready to leave, Mom got very anxious so the aide would have to distract her.

Mom loved to sing in choir all her life and professionally so when it was time to sing old time songs or hymns, Mom enjoyed doing that because "For the Moment", part of the brain remembers certain things. They had craft time and would have entertainers come in also. The local school children would come in their costumes and sing songs on Halloween. A band would come and play patriotic songs and the residents had a picnic outside on the patio for 4th of July week.

We would tell Mom's cna that we needed her to have special clothes on (which I had brought from home) if we were going to take her somewhere special on a certain day. They would make sure she was dressed and ready to go. Note: we washed her clothes every week. You could pay to have the clothes washed.

One day I was putting "rouge" on Mom's cheeks and said: "Mom, you have hard cheeks" and "For the Moment", she laughed.

It was getting harder and harder for her to get into our car. She could not lift her legs up as she was getting much weaker. She loved going to our home. Our last visit to the eye Doctor, Mom was anxious and we knew that taking her out was getting too hard on her.

On her 91st birthday, the residents sang HAPPY BIRTHDAY to her. "For the Moment", after they sang she said: "You all mean so much to me". When we took her to our house for her 91st birthday with our family a few days later, we told her all her great-grandchildren will be there. "FOR THE MOMENT", she replied: "But I won't be able to hold all of them at one time!" She made us smile!

Almost 1 1/2 years since she had her stroke, something was happening to her again. We were not sure exactly what was happening to her and then we got a call from the nurse and she said they were taking Mom to the hospital.

After three days and all the tests again, the Doctor talked to us and said that there was a lot of things happening to Mom's body. She was in a lot of pain. Her whole body was starting to shut down. Because Mom had a living will, the Doctor asked us: "What to you want us to do-Keep her comfortable?"

We had heard those words once before with Chuck's Dad. He had cancer and when the Doctor told us he was going to die, he said: "What do you want us to do? Keep him comfortable?' Dad died just a dew days later.

We brought Mom back to Orchard Court and the "HOSPICE" nurse took over and had instructions on how to treat Mom. The next day they had Mom all dressed up—hair done and she looked good, sitting up in a wheel chair in the dining room. We were amazed. She was even "talking a little". Well, where do we go from here? We wondered if she was getting better again.

Then the days and weeks to come were getting harder and harder for her. Now she was bed ridden and getting weaker and weaker. We would come each day and sit by her side. Chuck brought our CD player and we played Mom's favorite Hymns and sang some of them to her. Our children and their spouses came and sat with us, too.

As of this writing, there is a special group of people associated with Hospice who bring their harp or violin and play some music that is soothing to the ear and is comforting "For the Moment", for your loved one and for the whole family.

One day the Hospice nurse said: "You can talk to her. She can really hear you."

Each night before we left I would tell her "THANK YOU" for our children and grandchildren. I would name them all to her. I would thank her for all she taught me. I would thank her for being the best wife, mother, mother-in-law, grandmother, great grandmother, aunt, great aunt, friend and a beautiful Christian woman.

I would tell her "THANK YOU" for raising a WONDERFUL SON, CHUCK, WHO HAS BEEN MY WONDERFUL HUSBAND.

Each night we left her, we would kiss her good night and thanked God for her precious life. In the early morning after we had gone to bed, we got the call from the Hospice Nurse that Mom had died.

The twenty minute ride to Covenant Village seemed very long. We walked into Mom's room and there was a "red rose" on her bed and a "glow" in her room surrounded by pictures of "LOVE" of her family and drawings from her grandchildren and great-grandchildren for their "APPLE-MAE".

It was very hard saying "Good Bye" to our Mom!

We were at PEACE knowing we had done EVERYTHING we could for our Mom at 91 years old.

THE COST OF FULL CARE

Most older Americans are covered by Medicare and some have additional insurance, but both are limited. A long-term care insurance plan can help keep your loved one in their home for a few years with caregivers. My sister has done this for her Mother-in-law for over 3 years now and it does work.

When we moved Mom into her apartment at Northbrook Covenant Village "their fee" was a one time non-refundable fee depending on the size of the apartment, or duplex. You then pay a monthly fee for dining and maintenance, etc. Their fees are a little different now as they have wonderful new modern buildings added to the rest of the village.

Northbrook Covenant Village takes care of you through every stage of aging.

If you need assistance as you age they have "Assisted Living" apartments when the need comes with a little more care from nurses and cna's. Those fees become more expensive depending on your needs.

The "Full Care" units are a lot more money. With a room mate the cost could be up to $8,000 per month. When the patient's money is gone Medicaid takes over.

When I was first married in the mid 60's, our Women's group from our church went to a place called "DUNNING" in Chicago. At that time it was known as the Cook County Insane Asylum. We went to serve coffee and dessert to the women living there. It was one of the most saddest places I have ever been to and felt terrible for the women that had "lost their minds", as they use to say in those days. It was in a drab, cold, dark room and the women would just walk around and say "their family was coming to get them".

Some older people today still talk about people "losing their mind" and that is what some people said about our Mom. Thank Heaven we are recognizing the fact that we are doing much more research for ALZHEIMER'S DISEASE today. We have wonderful facilities with caring people to help take care of them.

There are a lot more Senior Citizens Retirement Communities and "Memory Care" facilities being built to satisfy the needs in the coming years because we are living longer.

To understand the fees you really have to talk with someone in the Retirement Communities as every person's needs are different.

PREVENTION

What can we do to prevent the disease?

Scientists know that Alzheimer's disease damages and kills brain cells.

Stay active: You can walk, run, swim, do aerobics or any exercise which may prevent or at least delay the onset of Alzheimer's Disease and even the forgetfulness often associated with normal aging. You're getting more blood and oxygen to the brain.

Control your blood sugar. A study recently published in the journal "Neurology" showed that people with diabetes are twice as likely to develop Alzheimer's as people with normal glucose levels. That's because high blood sugar and insulin resistance may lead to complications that could harm brain cells directly or damage the blood vessels that bring oxygen and nutrients to the brain.

Have your cholesterol checked. Scientists in Japan discovered that people who have high cholesterol levels were more likely to have markers for Alzheimer's in the brain called plaques compared with people who have normal or lower cholesterol. Another reason to watch your cholesterol: Conditions that damage the heart of blood vessels, including high cholesterol, high blood pressure and heart disease, appear to increase Alzheimer's risk.

If you start to have some symptoms of forgetting, you can ask your Doctor for a Brain Test to see if you have the start of Alzheimer's.

Mom had knee pain and finally had her knee replacement when she was older. Before that, because of her knee pain she did not do a lot of walking or exercising. When she had her knee replacement the other knee started to hurt but she never wanted to go through that surgery again. It was hard for her to walk around the block. You have to keep exercising to keep your mind active.

LIVING WILL

In 2010, we received our quarterly Township newsletter. The "Notes from the Nurse" stated that her Dad died on Jan 20, 2010—He was 82. He had numerous medical problems including dementia and heart failure. "Even though my Father was unable to tell us what he wanted toward the end of his days, we knew how to proceed."

Her Dad wrote advanced directions five years before. These papers were written with the help of an attorney. The Living Will spelled out his medical wishes for all to follow if he became incapacitated. He assigned health care proxy. A health care proxy is also called durable power of attorney for health care.

The nurse said her Father gave her the "GIFT" of knowing what to do when her time comes.

We were glad that our Mom had a "Living Will" signed by her.

We never thought about being a caregiver. We never thought anything could happen to our Mom, until one day she could not remember.

There are tests today that a Doctor can do to determine what is happening to the brain. Some people detect that they are forgetting but want to still be on their own until they no longer can take care of themselves. Every situation is different. Every person is different. Every family is different.

You must take one day at a time. You must be prepared and you must be strong. Faith was a very important part of all of our lives. We prayed each day that God would guide us through all that we had to do to take care of our Mom.

As we look back at how we helped our Mom, we know we did the best we could with her. We have NO GUILTY FEELINGS. We loved her like she loved us. Our Children and Grandchildren were wonderful with her and made sure they always went to see her. SHE LOVED ALL OF US AND WE LOVED HER.